ESCAPING THE SILENT KILLER

Charles J. Boudreaux

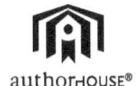

authorHOUSE®

AuthorHouse™
1663 Liberty Drive, Suite 200
Bloomington, IN 47403
www.authorhouse.com
Phone: 1-800-839-8640

First published by AuthorHouse 3/31/2009

ISBN: 978-1-4389-5305-2 (sc)

Printed in the United States of America
Bloomington, Indiana

This book is printed on acid-free paper.

DEDICATION

This journal, a chronicle, is dedicated to recovering patients struggling through long term rehabilitation. This endeavor, to which I can attest, will succeed if a positive attitude, self-confidence, and family support is maintained.

ACKNOWLEDGMENT

To my wife, Joey, whose love, sacrifice and strength has given me so much of herself these past five years. To my family and friends whose support and encouragement helped bring me from questionable health and uncertainties to a promising recovery. To those whose interest in this subject matter, and the knack for organizing, helped to make ESCAPING THE SILENT KILLER much of what it tells.

PREFACE

ESCAPING THE SILENT KILLER critiques the many aspects of dealing with a stroke and the years following. It speaks to the many periods of depression, along with the contrasting moments of gratification throughout the many days of participation in structured rehabilitation programs.

INTRODUCTION

Courage, Determination and Love

My stepfather, my dad, Charles Boudreaux, is going to try and prepare you to better understand and cope with this devastating illness by sharing what he has learned over the last five years. You will understand, and become aware of, the warning signs so as to facilitate seeking treatment sooner, perhaps the single most important action you can take to minimize the overall effect of a stroke. You will learn about the surprising sudden onset of, and long lasting, debilitating effects of even a minor stroke. But what you will learn most about a stroke from this treatise is how to deal with it on a daily basis.

More than anything else, it takes absolute commitment from you, your family, and true friends, to continue the fight toward recovery to the fullest possible degree. The fight is for control of your body, of course, but also for the health of your mind. There are few temptations stronger than the thought of just giving in to an insidious and ever present foe with seemingly overwhelming odds in his favor. Recovering from a stroke takes the fiercest determination one can muster.

Charlie will continue working to recover from the effects of his stroke for the rest of his life because he doesn't know how to give in. He will fight any way he can because he is not afraid of failure; he doesn't recognize the word. If one method of treatment does not work for him it is simply time to try another way. Most importantly, he has the lion's heart necessary for this huge battle because of the storehouse of love that dwells within him: love for his God, his family, his friends, and his life. Love that he has practiced sharing for a lifetime; love that now comes back to him to help in any way possible.

It is merely another testament to the way he lives his life that Charlie has worked to transform the extreme frustration of what is arguably his single most troubling life experience into something positive for you and me. In doing so, he is advancing his own fight for complete recovery.

Dance on, Dad !!! -- Kyle J.

ESCAPING THE SILENT KILLER

This writing serves as a timeline documenting a five year period of intensive rehabilitation and accompanying periods of enthusiasm and frustration following a stroke. Its purpose is not to solicit sympathy, but promote self-motivation, patience, and determination--all in an attempt to successfully obtain complete recovery--my primary goal. Throughout my life, I have considered good health and physical fitness to be paramount if one is to succeed in enjoying a full happy life. To do so, I maintained a rigorous exercise program supported by a sensible diet. Being a seventy-four year old male, I felt I was in reasonably good physical condition, but that was not my fate. On May 16, 1999, I suffered a stroke and immediately my life changed; so began my journey to ESCAPE THE SILENT KILLER.

A stroke is a sudden disruption of blood flow to the brain that occurs when a blood vessel bursts or is clogged. When this takes place, brain cells in the immediate area of blood flow are killed and these cells then set off a chain reaction that endangers other brain cells in the surrounding tissue. When brain cells die, one's control of his abilities directed by the affected cells is lost. These may include degraded motor skills, speech and memory loss. The specific abilities lost depend on where in the brain the stroke occurs and the magnitude of the stroke. A stroke is the third leading cause of death in the United States, killing nearly 160,000 people each year; strokes occur every forty- five seconds with a fatality every three minutes. It is amazing, that considering these statistics, fewer than 3% of the adult population cannot name a single early warning sign of a stroke. It is no wonder that strokes are referred to as " The Silent Killer."

NOT TUNED IN TO WARNING SIGNS

As previously mentioned, my stroke occurred May 16, 1999. My wife, Joey, and I were on a weekend trip visiting my nephew and his wife in Lake Charles, Louisiana. We were invited guests to the opening of their Bed & Breakfast, Mockingbird Hill. The weekend was not a hectic one, on the contrary, it was as laid back as you could get. After touring the facilities and unpacking in our assigned quarters, we settled in for a weekend of visiting with our hosts and my brother and his wife, who were also guests. Except for a Saturday night drive into Lake Charles for dinner, the majority of our time was spent sitting under beautiful oak trees, draped with Spanish moss, located along a sleepy bayou. Refreshments consisted of a scotch and water, or two, each evening prior to dinner and a couple of beers during the course of the day. In retrospect, this did not seem to be a setting conducive for causing a stroke, but rather the perfect prescription for recharging our batteries while enjoying a relaxing weekend.

On the Sunday morning of May 16, as we sat at the breakfast table, I noticed a slight tingle in my left foot and some fatigue in my left leg. These were the only abnormal feelings I experienced, and I assumed that my left foot had gone to sleep. I thought nothing more of it and attributed this sensation to the fact that we had spent most of the weekend just sitting. This was not the greatest diagnoses. There were no other suspicious signs: such as, discomfort in the left arm or hand or distortion of vision or speech, all tell tale signs of a stroke in progress.

Had I had additional corroborating symptoms and been more knowledgeable about strokes, I could have sought treatment at the nearby Lake Charles Hospital. The drug t-PA, a tissue plasminogen activator that links the number of cells that die after an ischemic stroke, could have been administered. This treatment is successful only when given within three hours of a stroke in progress and it can minimize the crippling that usually occurs.

We packed the car, said our goodbyes, and began the trip back to Houston about 11 A.M. My left foot was still tingling, yet I felt no reason not to make the three hour drive home. Once seated in the car, the tingling sensation actually seemed to subside. There still were no signs, with which I was familiar, to indicate a stroke was in progress. It was only when we arrived home at about 2 P.M., as I tried to get out of the car, that I discovered I had no control or strength in my left leg and foot. Observing my condition, Joey immediately drove me to the Memorial Hermann Hospital's Emergency Room.

Upon our arrival, a quick check of vital signs showed my blood pressure to be 245/120. The hospital staff immediately called in a neurologist and cardiologist for consultation. They ordered an EKG, chest X-Ray, and Cat-Scan to determine if there was bleeding or clotting in the brain. The Cat-Scan showed no bleeding had occurred, but did indicate a lack of blood supply to the right side of the brain just above my ear. The stroke was then classified as Ischemic. It was assumed that a blood vessel became narrowed, or clogged, slowing, or completely cutting off, the blood supply to neighboring brain cells. The Cat-Scan depicted evidence of three color variations of cells; the lightest coming from the stroke still in progress.

Once it was determined that bleeding was not occurring, Heperin, a strong blood thinner, was administered. Caution was taken so as not to lower my blood pressure too quickly or too low. The neurologist began by asking if I was experiencing any headache symptoms or any change in vision or speech. He had me touch his finger, then my nose. He also had me take my left heel and run it down my right shinbone. These are the standard tests used to measure a stroke victim's motor control skills. Upon completing his examination, I was moved into MICU.

JOEY'S MIDNIGHT VISITOR

The following is Joey's account of an event which took place that night during her vigil — "The clock was approaching midnight when the nurse in charge of MICU entered the room, for the third time, insisting that I leave. She took my arm and lead me into the family waiting room. I pleaded with her to let me stay with you, but she said that you would rest better without the stress of my presence. She promised to alert me of any change in your condition. As I left the room I could no longer hold back the tears; devastation and fear had filled my heart. I had been seated only a minute when I felt a gentle touch on my shoulder. I looked up into the eyes of a dear, elderly man who said, 'Come with me, I think you could use a cup of coffee.' As we walked down the hall, I told him about you. We had our coffee and started back to the waiting room. Before entering, he stopped, took my hand and said, 'I would like to say a prayer for your Charlie.' With heads bowed, this precious stranger spoke to God, asking Him to halt the progression of the stroke, to give you the strength and will to persevere, and to bless our lives with continuous love. He escorted me into the waiting room, gently sat me down, and told me not to worry, my husband was now in God's hands. As I looked up, my visitor had vanished as quickly as he had appeared; an unexplainable feeling of calmness and peace enveloped me. It was then I realized I had been touched by an angel and knew that you would survive."

REALIZATION OF STROKE DAMAGE

On the evening of May 17, a physical therapist evaluated my condition, followed by a Physical Therapist Therapeutic Intervention. This continued with fifteen minute evaluation exercise sessions throughout the next day; it was critical that physical therapy begin immediately. It was during these sessions, as I struggled on a walker dragging my left leg, supported by the therapists and her walking belt, that I began to realize the amount of crippling the stroke had caused. I was in awe as to the extent of physical damage and deterioration that had occurred to muscle mass and the loss of auto control skills in less than 24 hours; all due to lack of blood supply to the injured left side. As atrophy began to set in, the crippling became more realistic and the thought of spending the balance of my life in a wheel chair brought tears.

TRANSFER TO REHABILTATION FACILITY

On May 18, I was removed from MICU and roomed in the main section of the hospital. There I was visited by the doctor who was head of the Rehabilitation Hospital. He, too, went through the standard tests measuring my balance, memory loss, vision, and speech. In conclusion, he recommended that I be moved to Memorial Rehabilitation Hospital. I arrived there by ambulance and checked in on May 19. The thought of being transferred to a Rehabilitation Hospital for an undetermined amount of time, not knowing what to expect, and worst of all, not knowing my chances of full recovery, was an eye opening, insecure time for me. The support and encouragement that came from the Johnson family, Drew, Kan Dee, and husband, DeWayne, who were visiting me at this time, made things a bit easier to endure. I called upon God for help and understanding during the many nights I lay in bed, paralyzed on my left side, wondering what the future held for me. In fact, a night has not gone by that I do not call upon Him for strength and understanding. I did not ask Him to work a miracle and make everything RIGHT overnight, but rather petitioned His guidance that He give me the strength and courage to do what I must to overcome this attack on my body. I am firmly convinced that IF YOU BELIEVE, ALL THINGS ARE POSSIBLE.

My stay in the Rehabilitation Hospital was from May 19 through June 16. Kan Dee made arrangements to spend a few days with Joey, her mother, for which I am most grateful. Kan Dee was at her best. She took charge in making over my hospital room into a place that was uplifting and cheerful. From our home she brought family pictures, displayed the many get well cards I received, and completed the home-like atmosphere of my room with a stuffed ostrich and a beautiful plant.

I continued on the prescribed medications, namely: Plavix, Norvas, Heprin, and a Clonidine Patch, a combination of drugs designed to control blood pressure and blood thinning. During this time, I was put on a major rehabilitation program. The schedule consisted of three 30 minute sessions per day of occupational therapy and three 30 minute sessions of physical therapy, with regular evaluations conducted by therapists. Electrical stimulation of the left ankle and hamstring was applied intermittingly. With total dedication, much work, and a little frustration, I soon became self-sufficient in the kitchen; capable of preparing myself a simple meal. I was able to take a shower, with the aid of a shower bench and shower bars, dress myself, so long as there were not too many buttons, and tie my shoes with some assistance. While these activities may seem routine to the average healthy person, they were activities that I thought I might never do by myself again.

FIRST STEPS

I attribute the progress made in my recovery, thus far, to occupational therapy, the therapist who directed the program, and to the Physical Therapy Program which focused on strength training, resulting in improved balance, stamina and walking gait. The schedules consisted of the same number of sessions and length of time as the occupational therapy. On June 7, as part of my routine evaluation, I progressed from the wheel chair to a walker. About a week later, with the assistance of my therapist and her walking belt, I stood up and walked with the aid of a walking cane. Those ten steps were such a rush! It truly was the highlight of the month for me. Seeing the smile on my therapist's face made the moment even better. I can not say enough about these therapists; the majority were young women devoted to their profession. Their attitude, patience, and constant encouragement give patients the desire and the will to face a full blown, highly intense, rehabilitation program. These young professionals did that and I owe them dearly. In addition, family members Kyle, Tracy, Barry, and Nikki took time from their busy schedules to lend support and encouragement. Such outward demonstrations of love and concern meant so much and helped brighten the questionable days that occasionally occurred. There were visitations from many of our friends during my stay in the Rehab hospital. The display of friendship and support expressed to Joey and me were deeply appreciated. They came with gifts of candy, flowers, home prepared Cajun dish, and a therapeutic rubber ball to assist in strengthening my crippled left hand. Included was a collection of political/Cajun jokes taken off the Internet, which helped lighten, for a moment, the seriousness of my condition.

RECOVERY GOALS

Personal goal setting is critical to the patient and important to the Rehabilitation Staff. Their scheduled evaluations measure the progress a patient is making to reach his goals. I had only one goal and that was to achieve one hundred percent recovery in six months. Based upon what has transpired in the past eighteen months that goal was totally unrealistic, but at that time it did not seem so, and I committed every waking minute to successfully reaching it. I went through weekly, and sometimes daily, self-evaluations seeking to identify and quantify what progress I might have achieved. The smallest improvement was taken as a positive, encouraging step toward reaching that goal. I used that day's progress as motivation to work harder the next day.

In my judgment, the most rewarding therapy is a positive attitude coupled with self-discipline, and is extremely critical in the early stages following a stroke. A major pitfall is one's own self-pity, but when avoided noticeable progress can occur fairly quickly, usually in the first few months. Of course, this is contingent upon the severity of the stroke. However, after that, improvement reaches a plateau and progress becomes slower and more difficult to achieve. If a firm and positive attitude is not maintained, disappointment and lack of enthusiasm toward recovery and the willingness to accept the current situation sets in. If this pitfall is avoided, and a healthy motivated attitude prevails, the patient will be rewarded with new signs of recovery. The recovery process continues until the next plateau occurs, and once more the patient's attitude and desire for total recovery is tested, again and again, until he has reached his goal.

IMPORTANT TEST

On May 21, I was given a Neuropsychological Evaluation. The test consisted of writing, reading, simple mathematics, color variations, memory, speech, and other tests of skills to denote if any brain damage had taken place. The results were positive; all faculties showed to be normal. On a lighter note, while reviewing the test results with the doctor, I told her that my speech affliction was not caused by the stroke, but leftover from my South Louisiana up bringing! I was also tested for automobile driving capabilities. The Rehab Center had a full blown automobile simulator that measured my ability to handle traffic conditions and judge my overall driving co-ordination. Part of this test included several unrehearsed traffic situations. Again, results were positive and I was given clearance to resume driving when I felt ready.

ORTHOTIC FITTING & REALITY CHECK

On May 28, Lone Star Orthotics, Inc. came to my room for the purpose of casting my left leg for a brace. This surprised me, in that I had no idea that a leg brace was going to be part of my rehabilitation. It was delivered to the Rehabilitation Center on June 5. The brace was designed to aid my walking by supporting my left calf and ankle. I found it to be heavy, uncomfortable and difficult to manage. At this point, another stage of reality was setting in and I saw no time in the immediate future when the brace would not be necessary. Again, another plateau, and again, I was faced with another test. It was then that my next goal was set; focus on regaining leg strength and balance. If I was to achieve full recovery, this had to be accomplished.

After a little more than three weeks of programmed rehabilitation, and continual encouragement from Joey, therapists, and a regular litany of prayers, I was released from the hospital on June 16, a month from the day I had my stroke. The Doctor / Director of the hospital, upon releasing me, said, "Mr. Boudreaux, we can't do anymore for you, but you should be pleased and thankful for what recovery you have made and thankful your stroke was not more damaging." Basically, what he was telling me was that I was now on my own and to have a good life! My response was, "Sir, that is not acceptable." I left his office more convinced then ever that there was much more room for improvement and my life was going to be better, no thanks to him!

RELEASED

Upon leaving the hospital, uncertainty and self-doubt began to creep in replacing the safe and comforting environment I had experienced for over a month. I had been surrounded by doctors, nurses, therapists, Joey, family and friends, but now I was about to go home and enter an Out Patient Therapy program and essentially be on my own. I had made up my mind and stated that I could overcome this illness. How could I do less, given the outgoing support from Joey and family? As I dwelled on this, I became despondent once again. Another plateau, another test, became apparent. I again turned to God for courage, read and re-read the many get well cards I received from family and friends, and gave myself a good 'talking-to'. This generated enthusiasm; I discarded my doubts and stopped feeling sorry for myself. It had been more than thirty days, but I was going home!

I AM AN OUTPATIENT, NOW WHAT?

The Out Patient Therapy schedule consisted of three weeks of occupational therapy and six weeks of physical therapy. I completed this schedule August 16. Included, at my own suggestion, was a three day per week adjustment session by our chiropractor. I regret that the adjustments have not made any obvious improvement. A week or so after returning home, Vickie and Reagan, our daughter and son-in-law, visited us for three days. As usual, their stay was a working one. Vickie cooking and Reagan doing the much needed yard work. Just having them with us for those few days was a great lift.

Another concern that surfaced was what impact was the stroke going to have on my family, especially Joey? I knew she was strong and could and would do whatever necessary to handle this medical crisis. There would be major changes to our lifestyle. We both felt, all along, that we had done all the right things to remain healthy, happy and looked forward to our December years. Subconsciously, a list of concerns crossed my mind and what impact might they have. Would I be able to return to my piano lessons? What degree of impairment would the stroke have on our dancing, our active vacations, family outings, and the volunteer aid to our friends in need? As expected, Joey met the challenge head on, taking charge and assuming whatever responsibilities needed attention. In other words, she made me her first priority. My welfare and recovery came first and it was all done with love in her heart and a smile on her face. If anything, there were times when she tried to do too much and that bothered me, but this is something she cannot help. Joey is tender hearted and protective of those she loves, and I am fortunate to have her. Kyle says, "Darn right you are, Boo!"

Yes, she has met the challenge. Her strength and love permits her to cope with my condition, however long term. Joey made the necessary adjustments in our life, took over responsibilities she once looked to me to manage. As a matter of fact, there were times when I reluctantly asked her to back away and let me do the things I was capable of doing. I suspect this was one of her more difficult adjustments. She has accepted the fact and the reality that I am vulnerable, that I can become ineffective and need to depend on her. The same would hold true, if the roles were reversed. This whole episode has made us both realize how easy it was for our full and complete lives to be drastically interrupted. However, we both view these times to be temporary. The life we enjoyed for twenty plus years shall return with a ROAR. I have attempted to maintain our current daily routine and lifestyle as much as possible prior to May 16, 1999. The fact that I am hindered by my leg brace and still have need of a walking cane, will not interfere with us doing things or going places we enjoyed in the past, so long as it is not detrimental to my recovery. At this stage in time, we have not missed much, only some fun dancing.

IT HAS BEEN THREE MONTHS

August 16, was the third month anniversary of my stroke. Doctors, family, therapist and friends expressed surprise at the degree of progress that I have been able to make. I admit that I, too, am pleased with the progress, but grow impatient. I can see the improvements made in the past 90 days when comparing my overall strength to what it was on the evening of May 16. I feel confident that if I continue to work hard, my goal to function without the leg brace can be achieved in the near future. The self-evaluations I conducted almost weekly indicate this, and my regular schedules of home therapy have also been successful. These sessions consist of exercises directed to building my left side: the hip, calf, and ankle. I am absolutely convinced that once released from a Rehabilitation Center, out patient physical and occupational therapy in the early stages of a stroke are a must. I am currently investigating the possibility of working with a private therapist. She is the wife and part owner of the company that made my leg brace. Her husband, who designs and makes orthotics, suggested that I secure a pair of leather shoes which he claimed would help support my foot in the leg brace. I was wearing gym shoes at the time. I have done so and the shoes do seem to help.

MONTHLY EVALUATIONS

First month following stroke and released from Rehab Center-June 16, 1999.

- Unassisted bathing, balance has improved but blood pressure levels need to be lower.
- Continual weakness in left arm, shoulder and hamstring, unable to move ankle, and sleepy tingling sensation continues in left hand and fingers.
- Mobile only in the wheel chair, weight loss approximately 10 pounds. Second month after stroke, and first month following release from Rehab Center.
- Began out patient physical therapy both at Rehab Center and at home. Sessions at Center consist of 1 1/2 hours 3 days per week and home therapy, 1 1/2 hours 4 days per week.
- Increased strength in left leg, arm, and hip; Increased use of hand weights during therapy, significant improvement in balance, walking gait, and an increase in overall body strength. The adjustments to the leg brace have improved ankle movement. Wheel chair usage has been reduced significantly.
- Tingling in left hand has moved down to fingertips and across knuckles. Cardiologists made adjustments to the medication to further lower my blood pressure. B.P. is in

range of 165 / 90, (still too high). Now able to resume driving.

Second month after release from Rehab Center

- Completed Out Patient therapy. Began arranging for a private therapist.

- Increased strength in upper left leg has allowed me to shower without a bench. The need of shower bars continues, primarily for security. Use of leg brace and walking cane expected to continue for some time.

- No changes in the left hand, tingling remains. Doctors insist this is a residual caused by the stroke.

- Our level of entertainment has increased: attendance at The Houston Club has become more frequent. Was able to attend the Boudreaux L'etoile Acadienne Reunion in New Iberia, Louisiana and I was able to fulfill dance card obligations which I promised to do while still in the hospital.

CARDIOLOGIST CONSULTATION and RE-EVALUATION

I visited my cardiologist on June 23 and July 21. The visits basically addressed my blood pressure levels and changes to the medications prescribed while in the hospital. To date blood pressure lowering has been the main concern. After several medication adjustments, B.P. averaged 145/80. Another visit on August 31, for a full laboratory blood work-up was done. On that visit, my blood pressure was not to the cardiologist's liking, levels continued to be in the 145/80-85 range. Norvasc, a diuretic, was prescribed.

Also, the last blood work-up showed high levels of Total Cholesterol and HDL; Cholesterol lowering Lipitor was prescribed.

August 30th, 1999--Time to re-evaluate my physical and emotional state. I began to see signs of increased leg strength. My left hamstring is firmer, yet flexible, and has helped to keep my leg from kicking out as much when walking without the leg brace. Foot strength and mobility have increased. Walking without support of brace or cane is becoming easier. I contributed much of this to an improvement in balance. My home therapy is geared to concentrating on balance and focusing on posture. I do home therapy at a minimum of four days per week for about an hour and a half, plus out patient sessions. My left leg and arm still show signs of atrophy, resulting from the stroke. The difference in size of my upper left leg is quite obvious. Also, quite noticeably to the touch is the difference in skin temperature from below the knee to the foot and to the left hand. Mentally, I feel I am doing fine. I detect no hang-ups and have accepted the stroke and how it has affected me. I strive everyday to maintain a positive attitude toward life and my present handicap, however, an occasional reminder becomes necessary.

SPIRIT and EMOTION

At present, my emotional posture is something else. Base case, I am an emotional person and I have been accused, justly so, of crying over the six o'clock evening news. I don't become depressed easily, but do wear my heart and feelings on my sleeve. Lately, situations small and unrelated to me have brought on tears and a heavy heart. For example, this morning I called a dear friend who was recovering from triple by-pass surgery. His recovery was on schedule and the prognosis good. Yet, the sound of his voice, the emptiness of his demeanor all affected me to the point of tears. Prior to my stroke, this phone call would not have had this impact. Expressions of love and affection from friends such as get well cards, telephone calls inquiring as to my progress or, in general, just showing interest and concern, all affect me emotionally. My nightly prayers become emotional and even at this moment as I write I am moved deeply. Church services really break me up. I am not sure why, maybe it's because I feel a little closer to God and He hears me better. Can this be the after shock of the stroke? I think it might be. It is worth noting that I saw some of the same emotional reactions from other stroke patients while I was in the hospital.

What I want to address now is the status of my left arm and hand. As I have mentioned earlier, I continue to have a tingling and some tightness in my fingers, and some of the same sensation in my left foot. To date, my hand and arm have not gotten much attention, only the few home exercises that I do involve these areas. I plan to discuss this problem in detail with my cardiologist. I do see signs of gaining strength, yet there are days when I become discouraged. I realize the stroke depleted my entire body strength to a degree which I don't comprehend and it will take time and much hard work to restore it to it's prior 5/16 condition. Still, after saying this, it is difficult to accept and becomes discouraging at times. A good example was a day just recently. Joey, sitting at my side, asked, "Are you tired?" Immediately, tears rushed to my eyes and I blurted out, "I am so tired of being tired all the time." Continuing, I said, "Every single thing I do takes so much energy and effort. Just to shower, shave, and dress saps my strength and totally drains me. Sitting at a table eating, or sitting in a chair turning the pages of a newspaper require enormous effort." Presently, I sleep about ten hours a night and become completely exhausted after trying to maintain as normal an active day as possible. However, the next morning, I feel rested and look forward to what the day holds for Joey and me. I would expect if there is a single factor that can discourage a recovering stroke patient to the point of giving up, it would be the high energy demands required to just get through the day.

Physical and occupational therapy, along with prescribed medication, all play a huge role in the recovery process. Yet, to my spirit, the most uplifting factors that aid in recovery are the periodical phone calls from our children and inquiries as to my status and needs. Such unexpected calls in the middle of the day, or late at night, press my emotional button but give me additional strength to face what may come next. These calls are so gratifying, knowing their lives are busy and full, still they make the time. I don't think I am different in wanting and needing assurance from the ones we love. I think this is normal even if a serious illness is not a factor. This need and want is certainly provided by Joey. Her love, encouragement, patience, and strength fill our home and her most recent get well card expresses the loving atmosphere in which she has surrounded me. The following is an excerpt from that card "HANG IN THERE, REMEMBER HAPPINESS WILL COME YOUR WAY AND EVERYTHING IS GOING TO BE OK," I must confess that was another emotional and tearful moment.

NEW DOCTORS AND CLASSROOM STUDY CASE

We have all heard the expression 'One thing leads to another' and here is a prime example. The orthotic specialist who made my leg brace, and who sees me monthly, was most insistent that I continue with more physical therapy. I had told him the doctor in charge of the Rehabilitation Hospital was releasing me, ending my out patient therapy. I asked if his wife, a physical therapist, would be interested in working with me. He said she didn't have the time to work with private patients any more since she was teaching Physical Therapy at the Woman's Hospital of Texas, but she could recommend a highly qualified therapist, whom I immediately contacted. He came to my home on Sept. 7, and following a question and answer period, evaluated me, measuring my balance, leg strength and gait. He asked if I had set goals for myself. I told him they were the same as those set in mid-July while in the hospital—total recovery, back on the dance floor, non-dependence on the leg brace. He asked me to reaffirm that my goals had not changed since making them in the hospital. My answer was the goals remain the same. After completing his evaluation, Robert was convinced, with further hard work, I could reach my goal to dispose of the leg brace and return to the dance floor. However, to his disappointment as well as mine, he was unable to take me as his patient, because of his present full time job with the county. He suggested two Physical Therapy facilities, which I immediately pursued.

Shortly after, the Physical Therapist, teaching at the Women's Hospital, called inquiring as to my willingness, as a recovering stroke patient, to demonstrate my balance and walking, with and without my leg brace, to a group of her students. The group was studying for their Masters and or Doctorate in Physical Therapy. I consented and the date of Sept. 11,1999 was set. I was introduced to the students, gave a short history of my stroke and what had transpired in the last four months regarding my therapy. Then there was a time set for the group to ask me questions, as to my life style and health status prior to the stroke, my working career and so forth. For whatever reason, the instructor didn't want me to pass on to the students anything regarding the period of time and level of physical and occupational therapy I had received. Each student was to observe me and critique my gait, balance and posture. Their observations were recorded, followed by an open discussion. The session lasted about an hour and a half, followed by more class discussion. The students' observations were collected for further study and grading. I was quite impressed by the eleven young ladies; no men in the class. I had to compliment them on their chosen profession, and said, "Being one who has been there and done that, I feel that I can speak with some authority. I hope you realize the impact you make upon stroke or trauma patients. Consider that the patient has been surrounded by specialists, doctors and nurses all doing their jobs, but not necessarily displaying the assurance and confidence a patient needs. Later, you come upon the scene and virtually become the patient's main contact and support. Your positive attitude and warmth lifts his spirits, you help remove his anxiety and you form the bond between him and his illness. Your constant encouragement gives him the strength and desire he needs to face his journey through long term rehabilitation." I thanked them and the class was dismissed. I don't know if the words did anything for them, but they surely lifted me.

A DIFFERENT REHAB APPROACH

I had a few minutes to talk to the class instructor regarding my situation, that being my need for another therapist and hoped she might recommend one. She not only had one in mind, whom she highly regarded, but also a particular Rehab Facility that I could attend as an out patient. The therapist practiced at the Texas Institute of Research and Rehabilitation [TIRR], located near downtown Houston. Upon my first visit, schedules consisting of three one hour sessions per week for a month, followed by one hour session per week for a month were arranged. After that, further sessions would be contingent upon my progress and the need for more therapy. My first official working session was spent in doing a detailed evaluation. It was conducted with and without the leg brace and walking cane. I was encouraged and impressed to see that this was done with the use of a camcorder. Until this time, past sessions were not put on film.

The sequence of therapy at TIRR differed from that of the rehab hospital. In general, I was given a better understanding as to what the program was to accomplish. I was encouraged to ask questions as we progressed, and told the program was designed to benefit me physically and mentally. Further, whatever progress I made, encouragement would be forthcoming when deserved. This made me realize immediately that this facility's technique was quite different from the rehab hospital's program. It spelled out quite plainly why I was there and that I was to focus on the exercises striving to do better each session if I expected to see improvement.

As I entered into my fifth month of recovery, I began to understand much better what my therapist was trying to tell me. I needed to focus more on my rehabilitation and less on the stroke. All the appropriate tests had been conducted to help answer the question as to what caused the stroke, yet after saying that, the doctors were not absolutely sure. All that was behind me now, I needed to move on and be more concerned about what was ahead for me. The therapist helped me to do this. For example, we never talked about the pre-stroke days; instead, we concentrated on the program and the progress I made toward achieving my goals. At no time was he satisfied with last week's progress, but more concerned over the progress he expected of me in the coming weeks. He continued to challenge me by increasing the degree of difficulty of each exercise regiment. The results were quite obvious as indicated by my own weekly evaluation at home. These evaluations were strongly recommended by TIRR and I could see why, the progress achieved, regardless of the degree, was rewarding and motivated me to work harder.

WATER THERAPY

In addition to the clinic therapy, I was introduced to water therapy. I worked out two to three days per week doing leg and arm exercises plus toe raises in my gym's pool which I had used prior to the stroke. This program was designed to lessen the effort required to exercise. The buoyancy of the water permitted me to do twice the amount of exercise for the same amount of energy. In addition, the water left me invigorated and energized.

RELEASED FROM TIRR

Today, October 25, I completed my therapy at TIRR. The five week session was successful and rewarding. My therapist again taped my walking, balance and gait with and without the use of the leg brace and cane. He compared this taping to the one he did when I entered TIRR. We compared the two tapes, looking for changes and improvements made in the past five weeks. There were noticeable improvements, especially in the increased strength and movement in the left leg, also, better balance and posture was noted. Soon after we said our goodbyes. I thanked him for all he had done for me and promised to drop in occasionally so that he could see my continued progress. I am sorry to say, as of this date, I have not returned, but I do intend to do so. I owe him an awful lot, and credit this therapist with putting me on the right tract to full recovery.

REALIZATION OF AN IMPORTANT GOAL

Six months after the stroke, I completed another physical self-evaluation, and I am convinced that I am getting back a little of myself. To support this claim, I find that I am gaining more patience, tiring less, and have a general overall good feeling about myself. I am pleased and proud to say that I have accomplished one of the three goals I had set for myself in early June. It was goal number two, which was to be back on the dance floor in six months. The occasion was October 16, the first dance of the 1999 dance season of The Lords and Ladies Dance Club of Houston, a club we have been members of since

1985. However, I must confess, I was not at the "Twinkle Toe" level of prior May 16, 1999. It was a great night for Joey and me. The night was encouraging and rewarding for all the time and effort spent in rehabilitation the past four months. Further, it confirmed my convictions that dedication and hard work in therapy would allow me to accomplish my two remaining goals. Since then there have been several other occasions to dance and each time I find myself a little more secure in the management of the leg brace. I only have two remaining months to accomplish goals one and three. To meet both is going to be a stretch, but I am not about to say, at this time, that I will not be successful. I have come too far to stop trying now. After all, IF YOU BELIEVE, ALL THINGS ARE POSSIBLE.

CARDIOLOGIST CONSULTATION FIVE MONTHS SINCE THE STROKE

On October 28, I visited my cardiologist; this was my third visit and the fifth month since the stroke. It was an exhilarating visit, my blood pressure had stabilized at a level of 130/80, heart rate of 73 and the best news of all, my cholesterol was lower than at any time since measuring it. The total cholesterol was 161, HDL-39, LDL-97, RATIO-4.1 and, TRIGLYCERIDES-119. The negative side, however, is that medication is still required. I guess we can't have it all. I do hope that in the future, I may be able to eliminate some of the medication by substituting exercise and diet. The cardiologist, pleased with the results, moved my next appointment to four months.

OUR FIRST GET A WAY

October 29th, Joey and I are in a Timeshare on Lake Travis, just north of Austin, Texas. This is our first time since the stroke to leave home on an extended get away. These are times Joey and I look forward to. Just the two of us doing what we want, relaxing and reviewing where our marriage and our love stands. The second week was extra special as two events took place. First, Joey and I were presented with another beautiful granddaughter, Taylor Rae Johnson, born November 1. Both mother, Tracy, and dad, Kyle, are the proud parents. Secondly, Saturday November 5, we attended the wedding of Bervin Mirtsching and wife to be, Sandra. Bervin is DeWayne's brother. The wedding was every bit of what it was claimed to be, big and beautiful.

The following is difficult and sensitive to talk about, yet it is part of this story and I feel must be addressed. It is common knowledge that medication for high blood pressure has a dramatic affect on a man's potency. This fact came to pass this week. Prior to this time, Joey and I had not discussed love making throughout my five months of rehabilitation. I subconsciously wondered how I would be affected, and I was aware that the normal urge had diminished. Joey, in her considerate way, never pressed the subject, and was leaving it up to me. I felt, that in the back of her mind, she was more concerned as to the impact it might have on my overall recovery. In my previous visit to the cardiologist, the subject was discussed and I was told that the medication could have some affect. While still in our condo, the cardiologist's concerns proved true. Joey and I discussed the matter and agreed that this was temporary and in time would correct itself. While we both were disappointed, it was a relief to get the subject out and discuss it openly. We felt there was help, perhaps from a neurologist, and we planned on pursuing that possibility. Sex is not an absolute must to keep our marriage whole and strong, but it's just another way--a special moment for a husband and wife to express the love each has for the other.

SETTING TARGET DATE FOR FULL RECOVERY

Today, November 16, marks the six month anniversary of my stroke. When looking back, the time seems longer however, I do feel fortunate to be where I am at this juncture when considering the seriousness of my illness. A month after the stroke, I chose to set six months as my target date to reach full recovery. Looking back now, I realize that was too ambitious a goal. It confirmed what little knowledge I possessed regarding strokes and the length of rehabilitation time required. However, I feel it was the correct thing to do at the time. Now, I realize that much more time and work will be required, and it was important that another target date be set, based upon what I had learned the previous six months. It was critical that I continue challenging myself otherwise I could become satisfied with my present status of recovery. I was convinced that what progress had been achieved was directly related to my striving to reach the goal I had set for myself six months ago.

On my last visit to the cardiologist, I complained of the continual tingling in my left hand and the heaviness in my upper left arm and it was suggested I see a neurologist. In late November I visited a neurologist who was a member of the Memorial Hospital Health Care Group and was the attending physician in the emergency room the day of my stroke. He reviewed my file, including the medications, blood pressure levels, and examined my overall condition. He felt the tingling sensation in the left hand and the heavy feeling through my left arm were attributed to nerve damage caused by the stroke and suggested further testing. On December 2, he conducted an ultrasound on the upper part of the arm and down the wrist and hand. The test confirmed his suspicion of nerve damage and prescribed the medication Neurontin, which was to be taken twice a day. He concluded that the problem appeared to be a minor case of Carpal Tunnel Syndrome, but the damage, in his opinion, was not severe enough to warrant surgery.

So where am I today? It seems like more than six months since I became ill and I feel that my patience is wearing thin. Can it be that the almost daily routine of some form of physical therapy has become boring? COULD THIS BE ANOTHER TEST? If this is the case, I must make myself aware of this situation and not allow myself to succumb to anything less than what has been prescribed for me to do. I must maintain my firm faith that patience and dedication to a rigorous therapy program brought me to where I am today. On December IS, seven months following the stroke, I attempted to do a major self evaluation. I felt it was critical that I do a reasonably good review of my overall state at this time.

SEVENTH MONTH SELF-EVALUATION

- Handicapped aids such as wheel chair, walker, and cane have been partially retired.

- Weekly sessions at Rehab Center have been completed, and now engaged in water therapy three days per week.

- Began lightweight exercises at the gym. Electrical stimulation conducted daily on left leg. Specific leg exercises to control leg lifts have greatly improved, such that at home, I walk without the leg brace.

- My inner emotions have improved. I contribute this to my acceptance of the fact that I had a stroke, yet not willing to accept anything less than full recovery.

- I find major improvements in balance, stamina and no longer need the leg brace.

- An important factor in the status of our marriage has yet to return completely. Hope to again discuss this with my cardiologist.

- In the last 2 months, I have gained some feeling in my left foot and toes. Until this time the entire foot was numb and without feeling. I can now grip my toes against the floor and feel the surface. I am sure this improvement stems from the many toe raise exercises I do in the pool.

- With some disappointment, my ankle has not improved. It continues to be partially locked with only a slight movement in the up and down ranges.

- Much more time and some hard work still remain to be done in this area. The lower part of my leg has gained some strength making it possible for me to manage the leg brace better, should I need it on special occasions.

- After seven months, I find some gratification in the fact that I am now able to maintain a consistent program of physical therapy either at the Rehab Center, the gym, or at home. Still, my left arm and hand show little signs of improvement.

LOOKING FOR THE CAUSE OF EXTREMITY NUMBNESS

In late January of 2000, I discovered a magazine article on a study conducted by the University of Northwestern Medical School in conjunction with Stanford University. The finding was published on thirty four patients who suffered symptoms of Thoracic Syndrome ranging from numb fingers to arm fatigue. The source of arm fatigue and finger numbness was found on the auxiliary artery in the shoulder area. The injury interrupted blood flow downstream. Numbness in the finger can be one of the signs of the syndrome. Ultrasound examinations of the entire shoulder joint found what appeared to be a damaged blood vessel in one of the branches of the auxiliary artery. Surgery found an aneurysm, or bulge, in the vessel wall filled with clotted blood. The aneurysm was removed, the blood vessel repaired, and good blood circulation was restored. The article gained my attention! Could this be the problem with my arm and hand? On my next visit to the neurologist, told him that the medication he prescribed had not helped the problem in my left arm and hand. He suggested I double the medication dosage! I asked if he was familiar with the Northwestern / Stanford study on shoulder aneurysms. He was not; I gave him the article. He suggested I return to my cardiologist, in that this could be a vascular problem. I agreed to do so, but asked that he call the cardiologist. Shortly after, I visited the cardiologist and discussed the magazine article. I was not sure from his response if he was familiar with the study, or just resented me suggesting it to him. He reluctantly ordered an Ultrasound, taking into account the area from my upper shoulder to the tip of my fingers. The test was done January 24; the results showed good flow and no restrictions. This was good news, but disappointing. The root of the problem was yet to be discovered. Now what? What is going to be the next step?

LOSING THE BRACE, GRADUALLY

My physical therapist suggested that I start trying to go without the leg brace. He felt that unless I did so, my leg and ankle would become too dependent upon it. At the same time, he cautioned me to go without it only in the house and avoid crowded places. On January 28, I put the brace away and did without it for two days while walking in the house. I found little trouble, but limped more and my balance was somewhat harder to manage. My walking gait and posture became more difficult to maintain, still another crutch had been partially put aside! On the third day of going brace free, I became more fatigued and at the end of the day, swelling in the left ankle and the lower part of the leg occurred. Fortunately, following a night of rest, the swelling dissipated. I was not only going brace free in the house, but began to venture into some public places: grocery stores, the library and post office. I credit this big step to having gained more leg strength, increased confidence, and the eagerness to dispose of the brace as soon as possible. It, however, required more concentration on my part as I lifted my leg to step forward. Along with this good news comes a bit of bad news. Since the stroke, I have had four serious falls, and several minor ones. I have to continually remind myself to be alert to obstacles or conditions that might cause me to fall, especially when not wearing the leg brace. What a set back it would be if I fell and seriously injured myself!

As previously mentioned, going without the brace requires total concentration as each step is taken. The bending of the knee and lifting of the foot are actions that come automatic to the right foot, not so with the stroke injured left foot and knee. As an example, on a recent night, I filled two glasses of water in the kitchen and proceeded to the T V room. About half way, my foot caught in the carpet, I went down, and the two glasses flew in different directions. As I fell, I tried to catch myself on anything within reach, but to no avail. I fell on my left side injuring my shoulder badly. Why the fall? I lost my concentration when looking out onto the patio as I walked by. Joey heard the crash and came to my assistance. After I assured her that I was fine, she FORBID ME TO EVER TRY HELPING AGAIN.

CUTTING EDGE CLINIC THE FLORIDA NEUROLOGICAL INSTITUTE

Neither tears nor prayers will go unnoticed. The whole subject of my stroke has Joey and me eagerly searching and praying for any kind of information pertaining to this matter. We think our prayers have been answered. Primarily through the Internet, we discovered a clinic in the state of Florida that deals with stroke and brain injured victims. It is owned and operated by a Board Certified Neurologist. I made telephone calls to the clinic requesting additional information. In addition, I requested names, telephone numbers, as well as addresses of stroke patients who had previously gone through the clinic's program.

Without exception, each patient I spoke to had only high praise and positive comments about the program and the success they personally experienced. Joey and I became convinced that this was something we had to pursue. I made the necessary arrangement, and we left Houston for Clearwater, Florida on March 10, 2000. My first appointment was on the fourteenth with an anticipated stay of three weeks. With great expectation, we reported to the clinic at the appointed time of two P.M. The reception room was bustling with patients of all ages, many were first time patients such as I, and others were participating in the program at different stages. We were welcomed by the staff, as well as patients, and soon became part of the family whose one common interest was to escape the silent killer!

It is a proven fact that no two stroke victims are affected in the same manner and will likely have a reoccurring stroke within five years. It is the clinic Director's contention that a stroke patient who has diligently adhered to the clinic's program has not had a second stroke. Therefore, each patient's protocol for treatment is designed based upon the degree of vascular damage caused by the shutting off or restriction of blood flow to the brain, bringing on various degrees of paralysis, speech impediment, visual distortion, or any combination of the above. The Director, with his staff of doctors, prescribes each individual's regimen of FDA approved vascular dilators. My program called for two dilators, Accupril and Dynacirc, plus magnesium, and .81 mg. aspirin. This treatment was designed to lower and then maintain a blood pressure level of 120-140 over 70-74. This level of blood pressure, with usage of the dilators, will dilate the damaged blood vessels and increase blood flow to the brain, permitting the body to heal itself. To establish my correct regimen of medication and blood pressure levels, daily clinic supervision using B.P. monitors, Ultrasound readings, Trans Cranial Doppler measurements, and physician consultations were done to reach and maintain the desired B.P. parameters.

We completed our third week of treatment. Signs of improvement, while small, were positive; it maintained our confidence in the clinic's program as we viewed improvements taking place in other patients whom we had gotten to know. This was encouraging and confirmed our decision to be a part of this new found treatment for stroke and brain injured victims. In this last week of treatment, the Director had enough confidence in my progress to have me put away the leg brace, and in its place add a lift to my left shoe. I have not worn the brace since. What a relief, what a red letter day! It was such an uplift to put aside this tell-tale crutch necessitated by my stroke; another goal was achieved.

I cannot over emphasize the importance of adhering to the prescribed schedules for the medications and meals. Both are critical and must be maintained to reach the maximum benefits and desired B.P. levels. Major deviations can cause blood pressures to fluctuate, defeating the potential gains of the program. As we became more familiar with the routine, and the required adjustments, we found it less difficult to manage. We completed the three weeks of clinical treatment, along with counseling, and planned to return home April 1. I feel that Joey and I, individually, will for sometime to come, review and evaluate what the clinic means to us, and how its success will impact our future. For me, it shored up my confidence in that total recovery may be possible. We also had located another avenue to help me escape the silent killer. The clinic stay put me back into an environment where I was again able to compare my disabilities to those of other patients. Yes, it felt right to be back among my stroke peers, talking to, comparing stories, setbacks, and disappointments; but most of all feeding off of their positive attitude. I can't say enough about the contribution Joey made throughout this trip. She once again defined the meaning of the term Care Giver. For without her caring desire and determination, this trip would not have met the success it achieved. As we drove the 1,200 mile trip back to Houston many thoughts ran through my mind. Would the near miracle we witnessed there continue at home? Would the degree of progress I achieved convince me that attending the clinic was the right thing to do? Could its success and my dedication carry me to full recovery?

BACK HOME WITH NEW ROUTINES

There was so much organizing to do once we arrived home. Schedules had to be set up for medications, blood pressure monitoring, plus exercise routines. I had to become aware of exposures to drastic changes in weather temperatures since both heat and cold have a drastic impact on blood pressure. Daily schedules of food, water, and other liquids were necessary to maximize the benefits of the large doses of medication. If a main meal didn't coincide with the medication schedule, a small amount of food became necessary. When considering that I was taking four rounds of medicine per day, a fixed schedule for eating was a must. It is quite obvious that these schedules and limits affected our daily routines, however, the results showed great promise.

After several months, my blood pressure approached the desired parameters, and my overall health improved. I exercised three days a week at the gym, plus home physical therapy. My left ankle and foot showed signs of further flexibility. My left hip, thigh, and calf continue to become stronger, thereby reducing my limp and the kicking out of my leg when I step forward. In addition, I required less rest and performed small jobs in and outside of the house. I am well pleased with the progress made thus far, since returning from Florida. To support this claim, Joey and I are getting out more, attending more dinner dances, and rejoining the ranks of our friends. It is on the dance floor that I can measure my increased strength and improved balance. Of course, the down side is the amount of medication I am required to take. This does concern us, however, we do feel strongly, that in time, a reduction will be in order as was confirmed by the clinic. In the interim, I have blood work done routinely to assure that there are no side affects occurring due to the medication regiment.

SPREADING THE WORD

Shortly after returning from the clinic, Joey and I invited five of our friends to our home who were in stroke recovery. We wanted to make them aware of what is available in the way of treatment for stroke victims; pass on the information and the experience we had gained in Florida. We were not trying to sell the clinic or give the impression that it was an overnight cure. One friend was very interested. Her stroke impaired her speech and partially crippled her right leg. She subsequently made an appointment to enter the clinic as soon as accommodations could be provided. Her three week stay and treatment was successful, but her overall improvement was not as dramatic as mine.

BEGINNING YEAR TWO

Today, May 16, 2000, marks the first anniversary of my stroke. Much has taken place this past year. It has not been a fun year, rather one of hard work coupled with prayers, tears, and much needed support from family and friends. I seriously doubt that without the support and the care giving love of Joey, I would not be writing this or be at this juncture in my recovery. As I become more knowledgeable and am experiencing first hand the capabilities a stroke has for destruction of the body and mind, I realize how fortunate I am.

As I begin the second year, I find myself pretty much on my own, with no supervised rehabilitation, or official goal setting evaluations. However, this does not make me apprehensive; I feel confident and knowledgeable enough now to follow the therapy programs and the means to evaluate my progress properly. After all, I have worked with physical therapist for over a year.

When I look back and see the progress I've accomplished in the last six months, I have no doubt that continued dedication, self- motivation, and hard work in the coming year will bring me to near complete recovery. This is a promise I made to Joey and yours truly.

On July 11, 2000, Joey and I flew into Tampa, Florida for a three day follow up examination and evaluation at the clinic in Clearwater. Since we were from out of state, we were strongly urged to return in three to six months post the initial treatment. We felt the return trip was critical; primarily to have the doctors re-affirm that we were on the right track in implementing this new treatment. The three day stay incorporated testing, consultations with doctors and staff, and review of the progress I had made in the past three months. During this time, adjustments to my medications and tests measuring blood flow to the brain were conducted using a Trans-Cranial Doppler. We were pleased to hear that all test results were positive. The increased blood flow was significant when comparing the new TCD to the one done during my initial visit, confirming that the damaged vascular system was repairing itself. The only negative finding was that my blood pressure levels had yet to stabilize and were not consistently in the desired ranges. The doctors felt this would correct itself in due time, if I remained on the prescribed program. In addition to the encouraging tests results, it was good to, again, establish our friendship with clinic personnel and the young couple who owned and operated the Bay Queen Motel, our home away from home. We met many new patients who were entering the clinic for the first time. With a feeling of confidence, encouragement and the sense of satisfaction, Joey and I flew home July 16. We were ready to continue on our recovery journey focusing on exercise, blood pressure, and regaining the lifestyle we had once enjoyed.

SUPPORT GROUPS

I spoke earlier of trying to get the word out regarding the Florida Neurological Institute. One outlet we found was attending meetings held for members of Stroke Support Groups. Joey and I participated in several such meetings. We were invited to speak about our experiences in Florida. These sessions generated feedback from the patients attending and we hoped our presentation might provide enough interest for them to consider the possibility of entering the clinic themselves. We later heard of four stroke patients who were considering the treatment. However, since Medicare refuses to pay any portion of the clinical cost, the expense may prevent them from benefiting from the treatment. It is our hope that in time, as the clinic becomes better known for its success, medical assistance will be forth coming.

PROGRESS AFTER EIGHTEEN MONTHS

November 16, 2000, a year and a half post "S" day, a good time for another self-evaluation. I have found progress to be slow the past several months. I was told to expect such periods when recognizable progress may not be obvious. But if physical therapy and positive attitude were maintained, recovery will advance to the next plateau. It was in a later evaluation, that I became aware of changes in feeling and increased strength in my left leg and ankle. I still limp, but my walking gait has become more normal and my overall balance has improved significantly. I am now experiencing short, sporadic, mild, electrical shocks originating in the left ankle and foot area and reaching up into my thigh. I feel that these recent new sensations are signs of awaking and repairing of nerve damage to the leg and foot. Another explanation of this phenomenon may be what the clinic neurologist, with tongue in cheek, referred to as "Brain Rewiring." With these improvements, it becomes critical that I focus continuously on my left foot when taking a step. That is, how to place the heel down first followed by the toe. This signal, which the brain had automatically transmitted prior to the stroke, now must be re-established or "Rewired." Until this becomes automatic, I must maintain my concentration and focus on my left leg as I walk.

WHERE ARE ALL OF THE ANSWERS?

If I have learned anything throughout this chapter in my life, it is the lack of knowledge the medical field seems to have regarding what takes place during the recovery process of a stroke patient. What is happening through the course of my recovery are occasional unexplainable feelings that occur in my left hand and arm, as well as in the toes of my left foot. I become frustrated due to the lack of explanations from physicians and therapists when approached for answers to such questions. I am aware that no two stroke patients are affected in the same manner, yet, it seems reasonable to me that some of the feelings that I experience from time to time are common and are experienced by other patients. I would like to get some kind of medical explanation as to what is going on within my body and brain. Are these good or bad signs that I am experiencing? Are not these reasonable questions to ask? I have asked these questions many times and I am yet to get a direct or even an "it could be" answer. My entire left side was completely paralyzed and most likely residuals from the stroke still remain. My hand and fingers are the most affected, and tightness in the knuckles and tingling in the fingertips have not worsened, nor has there been any improvement. This situation is becoming very discouraging.

As I enter my second year post stroke, I think about what is in store for Joey and me in the coming year. While my last self-evaluation showed significant improvement, it is quite clear that much more work is required before a full recovery is achieved, as well as a test of my patience. It will do well for me to keep in mind the warnings of my doctors and therapists. Unless I remain aware that progress comes slowly, discouragement and pity for ones self will settle in, and the patient may be willing to accept the status quo. This is a typical pitfall that patients must avoid during long term rehabilitation. At this moment, I am grateful and pleased with my status. However, it is not enough, nor is it acceptable! Let's bring on the coming year and see how far Joey and I will take it.

A MINOR SET BACK

It's a fact we humans go along in our daily routines assuming that our health will be the same tomorrow just as it is today. We fail to realize, or we just forget, how complicated the workings of our body and mind are. Without warning, sudden and unexplained forces can disrupt their normal functions. Such an incident happened to me in the early morning of October 11, 2001. Shortly before 1:00 A.M. I awoke with a terrible headache. I could not think of what might have brought it on, since I rarely suffer with one. The pain was located behind my right eye. I woke up Joey asking for something that might alleviate the pain. After taking two rounds of Tylenol, which had no affect on the pain intensity, Joey drove me to the hospital emergency room. The doctor on call was advised of my stroke history and immediately ordered a Cat-Scan and a spinal tap. My blood pressure remained in its normal range, which was encouraging. The tests results showed no hemorrhaging, another good sign. Then a headache medication was administered via an IV. I remained under close observation and was released about 4: P.M. with a prescription for pain and instructed to see my primary physician on Monday.

I not only made an appointment with my primary doctor, but also with my ophthalmologist, because I began experiencing double vision in the right eye. His exam concentrated on my peripheral vision and eye weakness. He concluded that the major cause of the problem was the weakening of the eye muscle causing the headache. Further, he felt the double vision would eventually correct itself. As a precaution, an appointment was also made with a neurologist. His exam was a bit more detailed and he was concerned over the possibility of swelling behind the eye causing brain hemorrhaging. He ordered an MRI and conducted the usual tests for short term memory loss, such as, word association, mobility and vision span of the right eye. He, too, agreed that the double vision would correct itself.

In our second visit to his office, he reviewed the MRI results with us and to his satisfaction the test showed no brain damage. He identified it in layman's term as a ruptured blood vessel behind the eye and gave no explanation as to the cause, but did rule out a migraine headache. He forwarded the test results over to my primary doctor along with his diagnosis. In time, the double vision did correct itself. My primary doctor agreed with the neurologist's diagnoses and prescribed a stronger pain medication should it be necessary. We advised him of our planned trip to Colorado for several weeks. He saw no reason not to continue with our itinerary.

In about five days I was pain free. While the headache incident had no crippling affect, it did have an impact on my overall condition. My energy level, once again, was lowered and on occasions I experienced some problem maintaining good balance. It was never determined if the headache episode was a derivative of the stroke or caused by something else. Could this have been a warning to make me become more aware that I can't assume there won't be other future related episodes in my lifetime? That's OK, for with God's blessings and Joey's loving care, we overcame another challenge. As a footnote, this headache incident was put to paper during our stay in Pagosa Springs, Colorado, October of 2001.

One concern the Florida clinic stressed was the exposure to extreme hot or cold temperatures. Exposure to cold weather for long periods of time can elevate blood pressures, while the reverse takes place in hot humid weather. The clinic could not stress this enough. Our Colorado stay put this concern to the test and thankfully we passed. The weather varied with temperatures ranging from the low twenties to the high fifties. We did not spend a great deal of time outdoors, but the cold didn't restrict our activities. My blood pressure, which was monitored daily, remained within the designated parameters. Had the cold forced my blood pressure out of the designed ranges, adjustments to the medication would have been necessary. We were told how to do this in one of our many instructional classes at the clinic.

TIME FOR A PROFESSIONAL RE-EVALUATION

On the drive back home from Colorado, the thought of revisiting a physical therapist came to mind. I had last attended a Rehab Center in September, 1999. I had improved a great deal in leg and body strength, and felt the need for a professional to evaluate me. I wanted reassurance that, with the amount of exercise I was doing, I unknowingly wasn't damaging my knee or other body joints. I contacted the physical therapist who had helped me so much two years ago. He would be able to compare today's evaluation with the taping done in 1999. I visited my primary doctor and explained what I had in mind; he agreed and wrote a prescription for the evaluation.

On the first visit with the therapist, much of the first hour was spent taking my past two year history and my time at the Florida clinic. He examined my walking gait, balance, posture, and the lift in my left shoe. At the conclusion of the evaluation, he recommended I do more work to strengthen my left hip. He explained that to eliminate the kicking out of my left leg, further strengthening of the hip was required. He also felt that the left ankle was still partially locked, restricting normal movement when stepping with the heel down first. These were the two areas on which he wanted to focus.

The Rehab program he designed consisted of exercises that would help strengthen my left leg. He did not see any signs of damage due to previous exercises. After six weeks, he suggested I try another leg brace. This brace was of different design and weight, compared to my initial one, and it would support my ankle better, reduce the kicking out of the left leg and would further aid in a more normal gait. It goes without saying that the suggestion of another leg brace did not sit well with me. I was forced to wear the initial brace for about sixteen months following my stroke, but through determination, hard work and the Florida clinic, I was able to abandon it. Now it was being suggested that I return to it. The therapist picked up on how the suggestion of another brace was unsettling to me. He assured me this was not a step backward but more of a final correction. He went on to say that this brace was designed to correct a particular weakness in the ankle. It was not intended to be worn full time, just another exercising tool for further strengthening the ankle and would likely prevent damage to other body joints. I have always and will continue to be open to trying whatever might aid in my recovery; January 8, 2002, I was fitted for a smaller leg brace. I assured myself that, with God's help, I would not wear the brace for sixteen months as I did the first one. After using the brace for a while, I found that it did aid in my walking. The therapist felt it was a support I should have for times when I am required to do some extensive walking. It was put to the test just recently when Joey and I visited several of our favorite antique malls. I did find walking to be less strenuous, and without question, the brace aided me physically, but mentally it was a downer--- it remained a crutch.

ANOTHER RECOVERY TOOL

Continuing to seek out assistance in the course of recovery, I joined a weekly yoga class. The instructor is a dear, generous friend who volunteers his time and energy to helping a group of fifty or more adults maintain body flexibility. The class focuses on attaining control and balance through a series of held positions, coupled with deep breathing drills. For me personally, this class remains a pointed factor in recovery. First, the body control positions have helped improve my state of equilibrium increasing my self-confidence, lessen the need for the leg brace, and further expand my outside activities. Secondly, the emphasis put on bending and stretching of muscles and tendons has aided in the repair of my atrophy damaged left leg.

MANY QUESTIONS ASKED BUT FEW ANSWERS

A bit of melancholy may be detected at this point, but I assure you it is only temporary. As of late, I find my physical progress to be advancing at a slower rate compared to the past six months. This is becoming a bit frustrating. I continue to attempt to analyze what is taking place with my left arm and leg, but with little or no success. I sense new and different sensations and when again describing these feelings to my doctor and therapist, their response is still vague and not assuring. I can only hope these new feelings are positive and are signs of further recovery. Can this be another plateau or another test I must face? Can it be that I am becoming too impatient or maybe just tired? Or can it be that I have become frightened that the reality of reaching total recovery, my third and last goal, is unachievable? Will I have to be satisfied with what recovery I've made to date? I am aware that the recovery process is not always linear and changes are not always in a positive direction. Only God and time will tell.

REHABILITATION CRUCIAL AND EXPENSIVE

I previously addressed the subject of medication, rehabilitation, and patient attitude which are all factors in the on going course of recovery for a stroke patient. What I have not spoken to is the cost associated with obtaining aid and financial assistance. Granted, some help is available for qualifying patients in the Medicare Senior Health Plan. The program reimburses approximately 80% of the plan's approved costs for convalescing, physical and occupational therapy, and some medication. Patients who do not qualify for Medicare coverage are expected to be insured under a private health plan.

When a Medicare patient's benefits are exhausted, he is released and treatment is discontinued, although, it may be obvious that further therapy could enhance his recovery. If he desires to continue therapy, it becomes his responsibility to make the necessary arrangements and assume the cost associated with the additional treatment; a situation we find many stroke patients in today. The patient, who is insured under a private health care plan, is faced with an even greater obligation. In either scenario, financial burden can become a major factor in the decision to resume therapeutic treatment. If the decision is made to end treatment, history has shown, that too often, progress in recovery may cease and the patient can become discouraged and depressed. Without the challenge that rehabilitation provides, the patient may be willing to accept his present state of health. Recovery will likely come to a standstill, quality of life diminishes, and eventually, he may require full time home assistance. Perhaps if Medicare considered extending the length of treatment based upon a patient's potential for further improvement, the extended treatment could very well allow him to become self-sufficient. He would be less of a burden to his family and a substantial savings to the U.S. tax payer.

In another area, where I feel Medicare's present health care program falls short, is in its refusal to recognize some of today's new therapeutic treatments that are available to stroke and brain injured victims. Patients are denied the opportunity to benefit from these advanced techniques, unless personal financial resources are available to pay for treatment costs. For example, after the maximum benefits afforded me under Medicare's guidelines, I was discharged, ending my supervised rehabilitation. I felt strongly that further therapy was warranted if my progress toward recovery was to continue. This decision was based on the degree of improvement I had achieved in my six weeks at the Rehab Center under Medicare coverage. I located a private clinic that had developed a new protocol specializing in the treatment of stroke and brain injured victims. I entered the clinic with the understanding that its protocol was not under Medicare's coverage and, therefore, I would be responsible for all treatment costs. Patients were informed that the clinic had submitted to Medicare, and other government entities, documentation certifying the levels of success it had experienced in the treatment of hundreds of its former patients. It was the clinic's aspirations that this would convince Medicare to consider putting the clinic protocol under its coverage. There are approximately 550,000 stroke patients in the

U.S. each year, and costs Medicare $60,000-$70,000 per patient. My three week stay at the clinic, plus two one week follow up sessions, cost me approximately $9,000. Advanced treatments, such as the ones from which I benefited, have the potential to save Medicare thousands of dollars and improve the quality of life for hundreds of stroke and brain injured patients. To date, no action has been taken by the Department of Health and Human Services. However, there is encouraging and positive information coming from the Florida clinic indicating that Medicare is currently looking favorable at paying some of the clinic's treatment costs.

ATROPHY AFFECTS AND IMPORTANCE OF EARLY REHABILITATION

The following table illustrates the immediate damage occurring to the muscular structure through atrophy following a stroke. The time periods show measurements of the affected leg and arm prior to and shortly after the stroke. Also shown are the measured benefits following early rehabilitation and the continued progress when long term physical therapy is continued.

LEFT LEG AND ARM MEASUREMENTS

Time vs. stroke	Thigh	Calf	Bicep
Prior to stroke	20 3/4	13 1/2	12 3/4
Two weeks after stroke	17	11 3/4	10 3/4
Seven months after stroke	18 1/2	12 1/2	11
Five years after stroke	19 3/4	13	12

The measurements show consistent improvement with greater advancement coming in the earlier time periods. The measurements taken five years later are encouraging and emphasize the importance of long term therapy, if recovery is to be successful. Improvements do come slowly and can become discouraging making it difficult for the patient to remain with the therapy program. As noted in the table, it has taken five years of extensive rehabilitation for my leg and arm to return to near the measurements prior to the stroke. I now have a better feel for when complete recovery may be achieved, however, I am aware that age is a major factor in the recovery process. I, also, realize now that more time and much more hard work is necessary.

SOME FINAL THOUGHTS

This final entry, May 30, 2005, marks five years and two weeks following my stroke. I've concluded that this is the appropriate time to review the state of my overall condition, and close this journal. I am concerned that if I continue with future entries of general content, the story will become repetitious. The three goals I had set for myself shortly after the stroke have not all been accomplished. Goal three, to obtain full recovery, has yet to be achieved, while goal one, to return to the dance floor, and goal two, to put aside the leg brace, have been reached. While I still walk with a limp, I feel fortunate and am grateful for the progress achieved to date. However, the level of tingling and lack of strength in my left arm, hand, and fingers has not improved significantly, making the time questionable as to when I might resume piano lessons. At the present time, no credible solution to this problem has been determined, nor has there been any form of treatment suggested. There are occasional days when frustration sets in and it becomes difficult to maintain a positive attitude; especially, when I lack the energy to go forward with daily exercise routines. Can it be that after five years the daily patterns of exercise, driven through motivation, are becoming more difficult to maintain? This is a possibility, but it will be overcome and will not discourage me from searching for, or trying, new techniques that may aid in obtaining my third and final goal.

The intent of this writing was to document the many facets a patient experiences following a stroke and how it might benefit him or her through the course of their recovery. First: to help the patient understand, that to be successful in overcoming his disabilities he and he alone is responsible for his recovery. Second: to help encourage his acceptance to a modified life style. Third: to resolve himself to complete dedication into long term rehabilitation. Fourth: focus on and maintain a positive attitude. Lastly, there are thousands of recovering stroke patients desperately awaiting the day when they can set aside their wheel chair, fold the walker, rid themselves of their walking cane, and become productive once again. May you be one of them!! It is my hope that these words bring inspiration to the many stroke afflicted patients in recovery and serve as a warning to unsuspected victims.

The benefits acclaimed by the Florida Neurological Institute have been achieved and further strengthened my confidence. My blood pressure is now stabilized, at a guarded level, permitting me to reduce the dosage of vascular dilators first prescribed. Most importantly, I have exceeded the five year time frame wherein the potential for a recurring stroke was viable. I continue to seek out new and advanced medical breakthroughs with quicker responses to progressive therapeutic techniques that will further aid in my recovery. Until such time, I will remain on my present journey. With hope and faith, I will - ESCAPE THE SILENT KILLER.